Quick Plant-Based Meals You Need to Try

Healthy Ways to Start Your Day With the Right Foot

The Green Solution

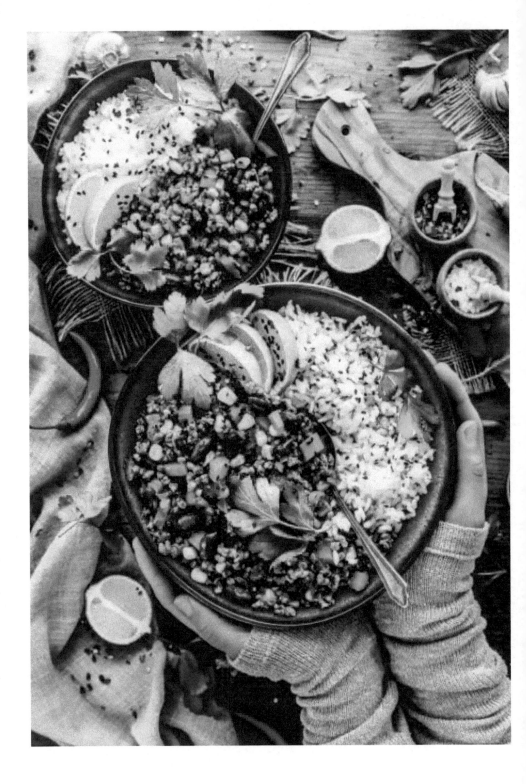

Table of Contents

INTRODUCTION

A plant-based diet is a diet consisting mostly or entirely of plant-based foods with no animal products or artificial ingredients. While a plant-based diet avoids or has limited animal products, it is not necessarily vegan. This includes not only fruits and vegetables, but also nuts, seeds, oils, whole grains, legumes, and beans. It doesn't mean that you are vegetarian or vegan and never eat meat, eggs, or dairy.

Vegetarian diets have also been shown to support health, including a lower risk of developing coronary heart disease, high blood pressure, diabetes, and increased longevity.

Plant-based diets offer all the necessary carbohydrates, vitamins, protein, fats, and minerals for optimal health, and are often higher in fiber and phytonutrients. However, some vegans may need to add a supplement to ensure they receive all the nutrients required.

Who says that plant-based diets are limited or boring? There are lots of delicious recipes that you can use to make mouthwatering, healthy, plant-based dishes that will satisfy your cravings. If you're eating these plant-based foods regularly, you can maintain a healthy weight without obsessing about calories and avoid diseases that result from bad dietary habits.

Benefits of a Plant-Based Diet

Eating a plant-based diet improves the health of your gut so you are better able to absorb the nutrients from food that support your immune system and reduce inflammation. Fiber can lower cholesterol and stabilize blood sugar, and it's great for good bowel management.

- **A Plant-Based Diet May Lower Your Blood Pressure**
  High blood pressure, or hypertension, can increase the risk for health issues, including heart disease, stroke, and type 2 diabetes and reduce blood pressure and other risky conditions.

- **A Plant-Based Diet May Keep Your Heart Healthy**
  Saturated fat in meat can contribute to heart issues when eaten in excess, so plant-based foods can help keep your heart healthy.

- **A Plant-Based Diet May Help Prevent Type 2 Diabetes**
  Animal foods can increase cholesterol levels, so eating a plant-based diet filled with high-quality plant foods can reduce the risk of developing type 2 diabetes by 34 percent.

- **Eating a Plant-Based Diet Could Help You Lose Weight**
  Cutting back on meat can help you to maintain a healthy weight because a plant-based diet is naturally satisfying and rich in fiber.

- **Following a Plant-Based Diet Long Term May Help You Live Longer**
  If you stick with healthy plant-based foods your whole body will be leaner and healthier, allowing you to stay healthy and vital as you age.

- **A Plant-Based Diet May Decrease Your Risk of Cancer**
  Vegetarians have an 18 percent lower risk of cancer compared to non-vegetarians. This is because a plant-based diet is rich of fibers and healthy nutrients.

- **A Plant-Based Diet May Improve Your Cholesterol**
  High cholesterol can lead to fatty deposits in the blood, which can restrict blood flow and potentially lead to heart attack, stroke, heart disease, and many other problems. A plant-based diet can help in maintaining healthy cholesterol levels.

- **Ramping Up Your Plant Intake May Keep Your Brain Strong**
  Increased consumption of fruits and vegetables is associated with a 20 percent reduction in the risk of cognitive impairment and dementia. So plant foods can help protect your brain from multiple issues.

What to Eat in Plant-Based Diets

Fruits: Berries, citrus fruits, pears, peaches, pineapple, bananas, etc.

Vegetables: Kale, spinach, tomatoes, broccoli, cauliflower, carrots, asparagus, peppers, etc.

Starchy vegetables: Potatoes, sweet potatoes, butternut squash, etc.

Whole grains: Brown rice, rolled oats, farro, quinoa, brown rice pasta, barley, etc.

Healthy fats: Avocados, olive oil, coconut oil, unsweetened coconut, etc.

Legumes: Peas, chickpeas, lentils, peanuts, black beans, etc.

Seeds, nuts, and nut butters: Almonds, cashews, macadamia nuts, pumpkin seeds, sunflower seeds, natural peanut butter, tahini, etc.

Unsweetened plant-based milks: Coconut milk, almond milk, cashew milk, etc.

Spices, herbs, and seasonings: Basil, rosemary, turmeric, curry, black pepper, salt, etc.

Condiments: Salsa, mustard, nutritional yeast, soy sauce, vinegar, lemon juice, etc.

Plant-based protein: Tofu, tempeh, plant-based protein sources or powders with no added sugar or artificial ingredients.

Beverages: Coffee, tea, sparkling water, etc.

What Not to Eat in Plant-Based Diets

Fast food: French fries, cheeseburgers, hot dogs, chicken nuggets, etc.

Added sugars and sweets: Table sugar, soda, juice, pastries, cookies, candy, sweet tea, sugary cereals, etc.

Refined grains: White rice, white pasta, white bread, bagels, etc.

Packaged and convenience foods: Chips, crackers, cereal bars, frozen dinners, etc.

Processed vegan-friendly foods: Plant-based meats like; Tofurkey, faux cheeses, vegan butters, etc.

Artificial sweeteners: Equal, Splenda, Sweet'N Low, etc.

Processed animal products: Bacon, lunch meats, sausage, beef jerky, etc.

Day 1:

Breakfast (304 calories)

- 1 serving Berry-Kefir Smoothie

A.M. Snack (95 calories)

- 1 medium apple

Lunch (374 calories)

- 1 serving Green Salad with Pita Bread & Hummus

P.M. Snack (206 calories)

- 1/4 cup dry-roasted unsalted almonds

Dinner (509 calories)

- 1 serving Beefless Vegan Tacos
- 2 cups mixed greens
- 1 serving Citrus Vinaigrette

Day 2:

Breakfast (258 calories)

- 1 serving Cinnamon Roll Overnight Oats
- 1 medium orange

A.M. Snack (341 calories)

- 1 cup low-fat plain Greek yogurt
- 1 medium peach
- 3 Tbsps slivered almonds

Lunch (332 calories)

- 1 serving Thai-Style Chopped Salad with Sriracha Tofu

P.M. Snack (131 calories)

- 1 large pear

Dinner (458 calories)

- 1 serving Mexican Quinoa Salad

Day 3:

Breakfast (258 calories)

- 1 serving Cinnamon Roll Overnight Oats
- 1 medium orange

A.M. Snack (95 calories)

- 1 medium apple

Lunch (463 calories)

- 1 serving Thai-Style Chopped Salad with Sriracha Tofu
- 1 large pear

P.M. Snack (274 calories)

- 1/3 cup dried walnut halves
- 1 medium peach

Dinner (419 calories)

- 1 serving Eggs in Tomato Sauce with Chickpeas & Spinach
- 1 1-oz. slice whole-wheat baguette

BREAKFAST

Homemade Chickpeas Spread Sourdough Toast

Servings: 8

Preparation Time: 15-30 minutes

Per Serving: Carbs: 33. 7g Protein: 8. 45g Fats: 2. 5g Calories: 187Kcal

Ingredients:

- 8 slices toasted Sourdough
- 1 cup vegan yogurt
- 2 cups pumpkin puree
- 2 cups rinsed and drained chickpeas
- Salt as per your need

Procedure:

1. Take a bowl, add chickpeas and pumpkin puree, and mash using a potato masher.
2. Then, add salt and yogurt and mix.
3. Now, spread it on a toast and serve.

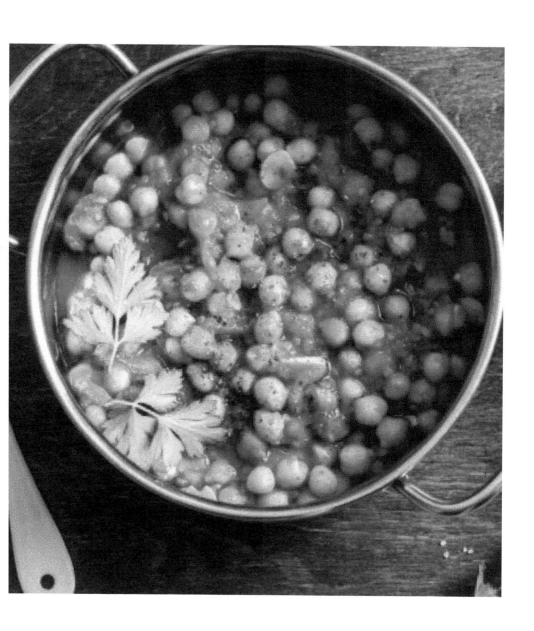

Servings: 4

Preparation Time: 15-30 minutes

Per Serving: Carbs: 55. 6 g Protein: 17. 8g Fats: 11. 8g
Calories: 398Kcal

Ingredients:

- 2 small diced Onions
- 2 cups diced Cucumber
- 2 tbsps Olive oil
- 2 cups diced Tomato
- 2 cups can rinse and drained well Chickpeas
- 4 tbsps chopped Flat-leaf parsley
- Salt as per your taste
- 4 tbsps Lemon juice
- 4 tsps Harissa

Procedure:

1. First, add lemon juice, harissa, and olive oil into a bowl and whisk.
2. Take a serving bowl and add onion, cucumber, chickpeas, salt, and the sauce you made.
3. Then, add parsley from the top and serve.

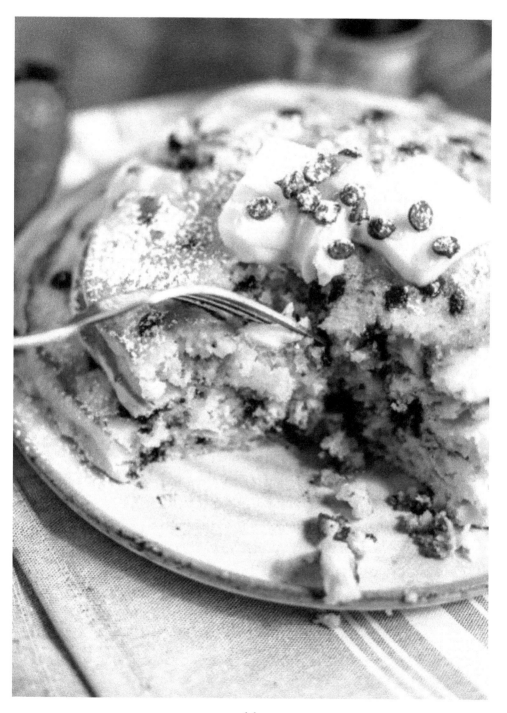

Homemade Chocolate Chip Pancake

Servings: 12

Preparation Time: 15-30 minutes

Per Serving: Carbs: 29. 4 g Protein: 3. 1 g Fats: 5 g Calories: 167 Kcal

Ingredients:

- 2 tbsps melted coconut oil
- 4 tbsps vegan sugar
- 1/2 tsp sea salt
- 500ml warm almond milk
- 4 tbsps chocolate chips
- 280g all-purpose flour
- 2 tbsps baking powder

Procedure:

1. First, combine together flour, salt, and baking powder and add in chocolate chips.
2. Then, warm almond milk in the microwave and add sugar and coconut oil, and mix well.
3. There should be no lump in the batter.
4. Now, combine together now, dry ingredients and the wet ingredients.
5. Then, add oil to the nonstick pan on medium heat.
6. After then, add 1/2 cup of the batter to the pan and cook each side for 3-4 minutes.
7. Finally, serve with vegan butter or any topping you like.

Amazing Toasted Rye with Pumpkin Seed Butter

Servings: 8

Preparation Time: 15-30 minutes

Per Serving: Carbs: 3 g Protein: 5 g Fats: 10. 3 g Calories: 127 Kcal

Ingredients:

- 440g Pumpkin seeds
- 2 tsps Date nectar
- 4 tbsps Avocado oil
- 8 slices of toasted Rye bread

Procedure:

1. First, toast the pumpkin seed on a frying pan on low heat for 5-7 minutes and stir in between.
2. Let them turn golden and remove them from the pan.
3. Now, add to the blender when they cool down and make a fine powder.
4. Then, add in avocado oil and salt, and then again blend to form a paste.
5. After, add date nectars too and blend.
6. On the toasted rye, spread one tablespoon of this butter and serve with your favorite toppings.

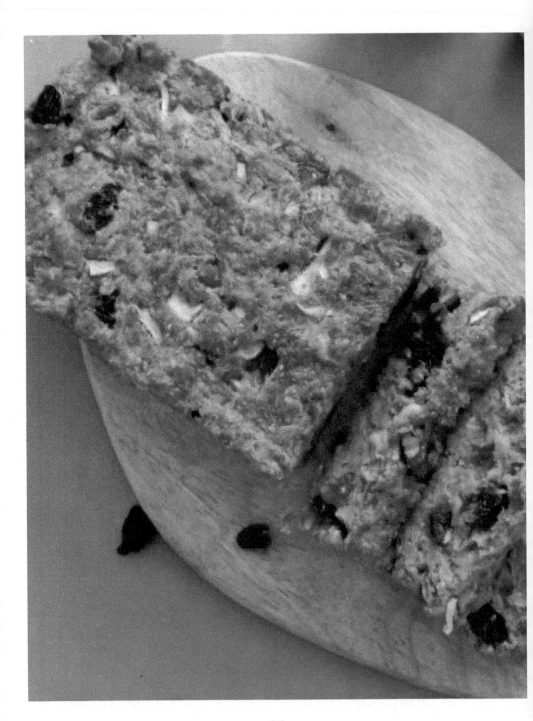

Delicious Chocolate & Carrot Bread with Raisins

Servings: 8

Preparation Time: 75 minutes

Ingredients:

- 1/2 tsp cloves powder
- 1/2 tsp cayenne pepper
- 2 tbsps cinnamon powder
- 3 cups whole-wheat flour
- 1 tsp nutmeg powder
- 1/2 cup olive oil
- 1 cup unsweetened applesauce
- 1/2 cup almond flour
- 8 carrots, shredded
- 3 tsps baking powder
- 6 tbsps unsweetened chocolate chips
- 1/2 tsp salt
- 1,1/3 cups black raisins
- 4 tbsps flax seed powder
- 1 cup pure date sugar
- 1/2 cup pure maple syrup
- 1,1/2 tsps almond extract
- 2 tbsps grated lemon zest

Procedure:

1. First, preheat the oven to 375 F and line a loaf tin with baking paper.
2. Take a bowl; mix all the flour, salt, cloves powder, cayenne pepper, cinnamon powder, nutmeg powder, and baking powder.
3. Now, take another bowl, mix the flax seed powder, 12 tbsps of water, and allow thickening for 5 minutes.
4. Then, mix in the date sugar, maple syrup, almond extract, lemon zest, applesauce, and olive oil.
5. Combine both mixtures until smooth and fold in the carrots, chocolate chips, and raisins.
6. Now, pour the mixture into a loaf pan and bake in the oven until golden brown on top or a toothpick inserted into the bread comes out clean, 45-50 minutes.
7. In the end, remove from the oven, transfer the bread onto a wire rack to cool, slice, and serve.

Servings: 8

Preparation Time: 55 minutes

Ingredients:

- 4 pinches of salt
- 3 cups unsweetened almond milk
- 1 tsp fresh lemon zest
- 2 tbsps fresh pineapple juice
- 4 tbsps maple syrup + extra for drizzling
- 16 whole-grain bread slices
- 1 cup almond flour
- 4 tbsps flax seed powder
- 1 tbsp cinnamon powder

Procedure:

1. First, preheat the oven to 400 F and lightly grease a roasting rack with olive oil.
2. Set aside.
3. Take a medium bowl, mix the flax seed powder with 6 tbsps of water and allow thickening for 5 to 10 minutes.
4. Whisk in the almond milk, almond flour, maple syrup, salt, cinnamon powder, lemon zest, and pineapple juice.

5. Now, soak the bread on both sides in the almond milk mixture and allow sitting on a plate for 2 to 3 minutes.
6. Then, heat a large skillet over medium heat and place the bread in the pan.
7. Cook until golden brown on the bottom side.
8. After that, flip the bread and cook further until golden brown on the other side, 4 minutes in total.
9. In the end, transfer to a plate, drizzle some maple syrup on top and serve immediately.

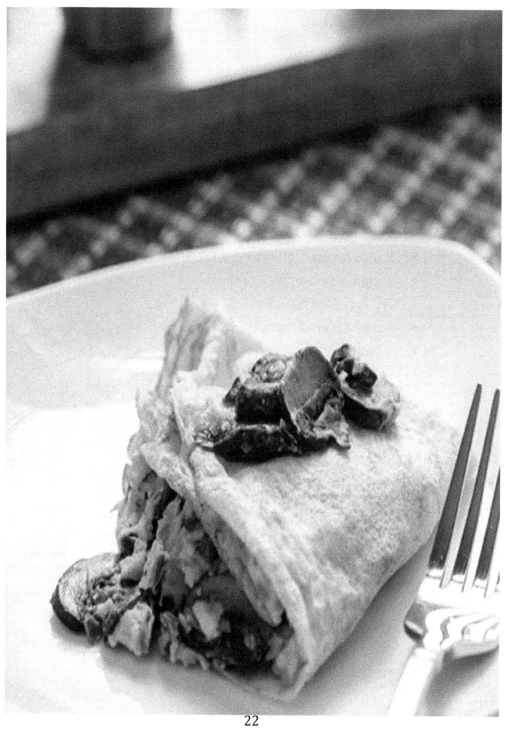

Servings: 8

Preparation Time: 25 minutes

Ingredients:

- 1 tsp baking soda
- 1/2 tsp salt
- 1 cup finely chopped onion
- 2 cups pressed, crumbled tofu
- 1 cup finely chopped mushrooms
- 2/3 cup plant-based milk
- 4 cups collard greens
- 2 cups whole-wheat flour
- 1/2 cup lemon juice
- 2 tsps onion powder
- 4 tbsps of extra-virgin olive oil

Procedure:

1. First, combine the flour, onion powder, baking soda, and salt in a bowl.
2. Blitz the tofu, milk, lemon juice, and oil in a food processor over high speed for 30 seconds.
3. Now, pour over the flour mixture and mix to combine well.
4. Then, add in the mushrooms, onion, and collard greens.
5. Heat a skillet and grease with cooking spray.

6. Now, lower the heat and spread a ladleful of the batter across the surface of the skillet.
7. Then, cook for 4 minutes on both sides or until set.
8. Remove to a plate.
9. Now, repeat the process until no batter is left, greasing with a little more oil, if needed.
10. Finally, serve.

Tasty Banana French Toast with Strawberry Syrup

Servings: 16

Preparation Time: 40 minutes

Ingredients:

- 2 tsps pure vanilla extract
- 1/2 tsp ground nutmeg
- 1 tsp ground cinnamon
- 4 tbsps maple syrup
- 3 tsps arrowroot powder
- 4 tbsps water
- 2 bananas, mashed
- 2 cups coconut milk
- A pinch of salt
- 16 slices whole-grain bread
- 2 cups strawberries

Procedure:

1. Take a bowl, stir banana, coconut milk, vanilla, nutmeg, cinnamon, arrowroot, and salt.
2. Now, dip each bread slice in the banana mixture and arrange it on a baking tray.
3. Spread the remaining banana mixture over the top.
4. Then, bake for 30 minutes until the tops are lightly browned.

5. Take a pot over medium heat; put the strawberries, water, and maple syrup.
6. Simmer for 15-10 minutes until the berries breaking up and the liquid has reduced.
7. Now, serve topped with strawberry syrup.

Servings: 4

Preparation Time: 30 minutes

Per Serving: Calories: 345; Fat: 12g; Carbs: 51.4g; Protein: 10.8g

Ingredients:

- 2 tsps salt
- 1 tsp baking soda
- 2 tbsps melted unsalted plant butter
- 1 tsp garlic powder
- 2 (8 oz) jar chopped pimientos
- 1/2 tsp black pepper
- 1/2 cup plant butter, cold and cubed
- 4 tsps baking powder
- 4 cups whole-wheat flour
- 1,1/2 cups coconut milk
- 2 cups shredded cashew cheese

Procedure:

1. First, preheat the oven to 450 F and line a baking sheet with parchment paper.
2. Set aside.
3. Take a medium bowl; mix the flour, baking powder, salt, baking soda, garlic powder, and black pepper.
4. Now, add the cold butter using a hand mixer until the mixture is the size of small peas.

27

5. Then, pour in 1½ of the coconut milk and continue whisking.
6. Continue adding the remaining coconut milk, a tablespoonful at a time, until dough forms.
7. Then, mix in the cashew cheese and pimientos. (If the dough is too wet to handle, mix in a little bit more flour until it is manageable).
8. Place the dough on a lightly floured surface and flatten the dough into ½-inch thickness.
9. Use a 2 ½-inch round cutter to cut out biscuits' pieces from the dough.
10. Now, gather, re-roll the dough once and continue cutting out biscuits.
11. After that, arrange the biscuits on the prepared pan and brush the tops with the melted butter.
12. Now, bake for 12-14 minutes or until the biscuits are golden brown.
13. Finally, cool and serve.

Healthy Easy Omelet with Tomato and Hummus

Servings: 4

Preparation Time: 20 minutes

Per Serving: Calories: 324; Fat: 20.3g; Carbs: 18.4g; Protein: 18g

Ingredients:

- 20 ounces silken tofu, pressed
- 2 teaspoons balsamic vinegar
- Kala namak salt and black pepper
- 1 teaspoon turmeric powder
- 4 tablespoons olive oil
- 8 tablespoons water
- 6 tablespoons nutritional yeast
- 4 teaspoons arrowroot powder

Topping:

- 2 medium tomatoes, sliced
- 4 scallions, chopped
- 4 tablespoons hummus
- 2 teaspoons garlic, minced

Procedure:

1. Take your blender or food processor, mix the tofu, water, balsamic vinegar, nutritional yeast,

arrowroot powder, turmeric powder, salt, and black pepper.

2. Then, process until you have a smooth and uniform paste.
3. Take a nonstick skillet, heat the olive oil until sizzling.
4. Pour in 1 of the tofu mixture and spread it with a spatula.
5. Now, cook for about 6 minutes or until set; flip and cook it for another 3 minutes.
6. Slide the omelet onto a serving plate.
7. Then, repeat with the remaining batter.
8. Now, place the topping ingredients over half of each omelet.
9. Finally, fold unfilled half of your omelet over the filling.

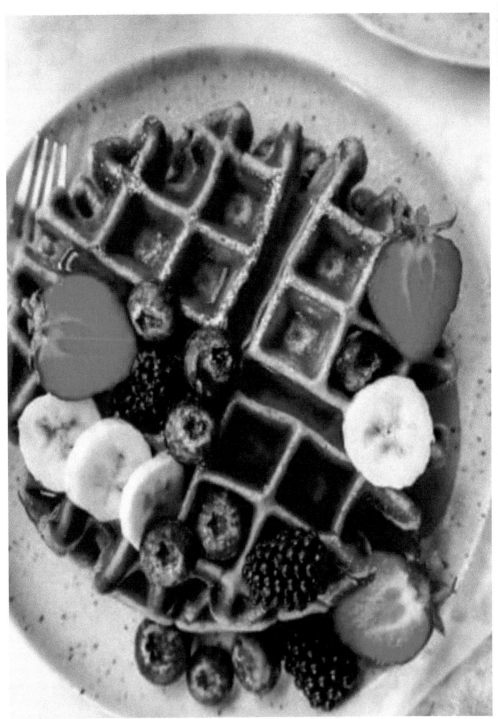

Servings: 8

Preparation Time: 20 minutes

Per Serving: Calories: 316; Fat: 9.9g; Carbs: 50.4g; Protein: 8.3g

Ingredients:

- A pinch of salt
- 2 tablespoons fresh lime juice
- 1/2 teaspoon ground cinnamon
- 1/2 teaspoon grated nutmeg
- 2 cups all-purpose flour
- 1 cup spelt flour
- 2 teaspoons baking powder
- 1 teaspoon vanilla extract
- 2 cups almond milk, unsweetened
- 4 tablespoons blackstrap molasses
- 4 tablespoons coconut oil, melted

Procedure:

1. First, preheat waffle iron according to the manufacturer's instructions.
2. Take a mixing bowl; thoroughly combine the flour, baking powder, salt, cinnamon, nutmeg, and vanilla extract.
3. Then, in another bowl, mix the liquid ingredients.

4. Then, gradually add in the wet mixture to the dry mixture.
5. Beat until everything is well blended.
6. Now, ladle 1/4 of the batter into the preheated waffle iron and cook until the waffles are golden and crisp.
7. After repeat with the remaining batter.
8. Lastly, serve your waffles with a fruit compote or coconut cream, if desired.

Servings: 6

Preparation Time: 30 minutes

Ingredients:

- 2 small white onions, chopped
- 1 teaspoon turmeric
- 1 teaspoon red pepper flakes
- 2 medium avocadoes, pitted, peeled, and sliced
- 1/2 cup nutritional yeast
- 24 ounces firm tofu, cubed
- 2 medium tomatoes, sliced
- 6 teaspoons sesame oil
- 6 cups water
- 2 cups stone-ground corn grits
- 2 thyme sprigs
- 2 rosemary sprigs
- 2 bay leafs

Procedure:

1. First, heat the sesame oil in a wok over moderately high heat.
2. Now, fry your tofu for about 6 minutes.
3. Then, add in the onion, turmeric, and red pepper and continue cooking until the tofu is crisp on all sides and the onion is tender and translucent.

4. Take a saucepan, place the water, grits, thyme sprig, rosemary sprig, and bay leaf and bring to a boil.
5. Then, turn the heat to a simmer, cover, and let it cook for approximately 20 minutes or until most of the water is absorbed.
6. Now, add in the nutritional yeast and stir to combine well.
7. Divide the grits between serving bowls and top with the fried tofu/onion mixture.
8. Finally, top with tomato and avocado, salt to taste, and serve immediately.

Servings: 6

Preparation Time: 10 minutes

Per Serving: Calories: 411 Cal Fat: 17 g Carbs: 50 g Protein: 20 g Fiber: 18

Ingredients:

- 2 tablespoons tomato paste
- 1 medium white onion, sliced
- 4 medium tomatoes, chopped
- 1 cup sliced sweet potatoes
- 5 cups vegetable stock
- 1 cup sliced potatoes
- 2 teaspoons lemon juice
- 1 cup broccoli florets
- 4 teaspoons minced garlic
- 2 inch of ginger, grated
- 1 cup red lentils
- 1/2 teaspoon ground black pepper
- 2 teaspoons salt
- 3 teaspoons ground cumin
- 1 cup sliced zucchini
- 1 cup baby spinach
- 4 teaspoons ground coriander
- 4 tablespoons peanuts
- 2 teaspoons Harissa Spice Blend
- 2 tablespoons sambal oelek

- 1/2 cup almond butter
- 2 teaspoons olive oil

Procedure:

1. Take a large saucepan, place it over medium heat, add oil, and when hot, add onion and cook for 5 minutes until translucent.
2. Meanwhile, place tomatoes in a blender, add garlic, ginger, and sambal oelek along with all the spices, and pulse until pureed.
3. Now, pour this mixture into the onions, cook for 5 minutes, then add remaining ingredients except for spinach, peanuts, and lemon juice; simmer for 15 minutes.
4. Then, taste to adjust the seasoning, stir in spinach and cook for 5 minutes until cooked.
5. Lastly, ladle soup into bowls, garnish with lime juice and peanuts and serve.

SOUPS

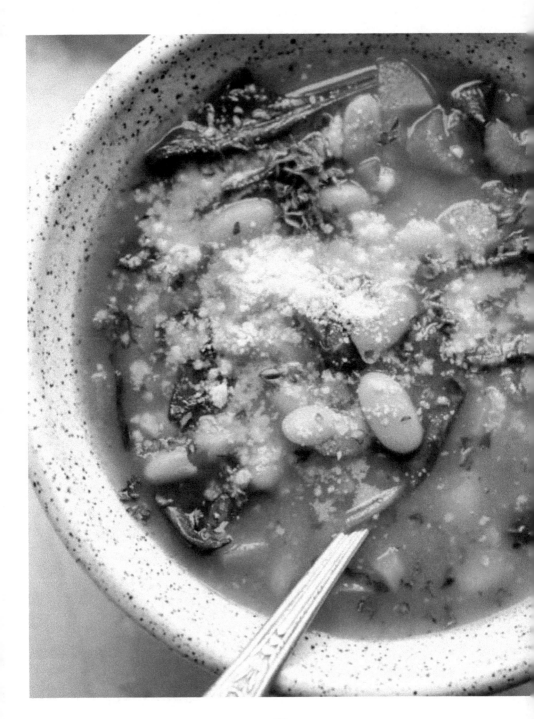

Servings: 8

Preparation Time: 5 minutes

Per Serving: Calories 111, Total Fat 7.2g, Saturated Fat 1g, Cholesterol 0mg, Sodium 8mg, Total Carbohydrate 10.4g, Dietary Fiber 3g, Total Sugars 4.4g, Protein 2.6g, Calcium 25mg, Iron 1mg, Potassium 170mg, Phosphorus 104mg

Ingredients:

- 4 medium onions, finely chopped
- 4 tablespoons olive oil
- Salt and pepper to taste
- 4 cups of water
- 6 cups fresh shelled green beans

Procedure:

1. First, heat the olive oil in a heavy-bottomed saucepan over medium heat.
2. Now, cook the onions until soft and translucent, about 3 minutes.
3. Then, pour in the water and beans, season to taste with salt and pepper.
4. Increase the heat to medium-high, bring to a boil, then reduce heat to low, cover, and simmer until the peas are tender, 12 to 18 minutes.

5. Puree the peas in a blender or food processor in batches.
6. Now, strain back into the saucepan.
7. Finally, season to taste with salt and pepper before serving.

Servings: 8

Preparation Time: 15 minutes

Per Serving: Calories 116, Total Fat 5.1g, Saturated Fat 0.7g, Cholesterol 0mg, Sodium 4mg, Total Carbohydrate 14.7g, Dietary Fiber 1.7g, Total Sugars 1.9g, Protein 3.2g, Calcium 13mg, Iron 1mg, Potassium 100mg, Phosphorus 105 mg

Ingredients:

- 2 large onions finely chopped
- 2 tablespoons chopped fresh parsley
- 2 cups macaroni
- 4 tablespoons olive oil
- 2 cups of water
- 4 large cloves garlic, minced
- 1/2teaspoon Italian seasoning
- 1/2 teaspoon garlic powder
- Black pepper to taste

Procedure:

1. First, heat the olive oil in a soup pot over medium-low heat.
2. Now, stir in the minced garlic and onion; cook and stir until soft, about 5 minutes.
3. Then, turn heat to medium; stir in water, Italian seasoning, parsley, garlic powder, and pepper.

4. Bring to a simmer.
5. Now, cook for 40 minutes with the lid slightly ajar.
6. In the end, stir macaroni into soup; cook at a strong simmer until macaroni is tender, about 12 minutes.

Servings: 8

Preparation Time: 30 minutes

Per Serving: Calories 57, Total Fat 2.4g, Saturated Fat 0.3g, Cholesterol 0mg, Sodium 98mg, Total Carbohydrate 8.5g, Dietary Fiber 2.3g, Total Sugars 4g, Protein 1.1g, Calcium 37mg, Iron 0mg, Potassium 249mg, Phosphorus 150 mg

Ingredients:

- 1/2 medium head green cabbage, thinly sliced
- 1/4 teaspoon salt
- 2 teaspoons dried parsley
- 4 cloves of garlic, smashed
- 2 large onions, thinly sliced
- 1/2 teaspoon dried basil
- Ground black pepper to taste
- 2 cups cauliflower, thinly sliced
- 8 large carrots, thinly sliced
- 12 cups of water
- 2 tablespoons olive oil
- 1/2 teaspoon dried thyme

Procedure:

1. First, combine the carrots, cauliflower, onion, cabbage, garlic, water, olive oil, thyme, basil,

parsley, salt, and pepper in a pot over medium-high heat; bring to a simmer and cook until the carrots are tender for about 20 minutes.

2. Then, transfer to a blender in small batches and blend until smooth.

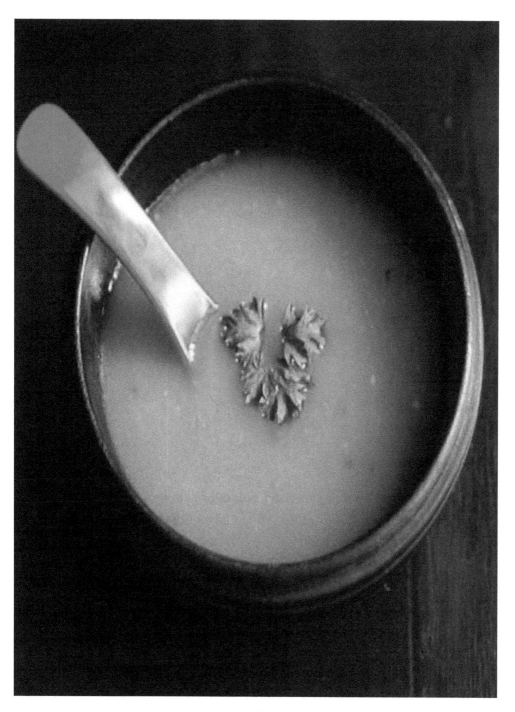

Servings: 8

Preparation Time: 20 minutes

Per Serving: Calories 169, Total Fat 17.7g, Saturated Fat 2.5g, Cholesterol 0mg, Sodium 81mg, Total Carbohydrate 4.1g, Dietary Fiber 0.9g, Total Sugars 1.5g, Protein 0.6g, Calcium 38mg, Iron 1mg, Potassium 140mg, Phosphorus 90 mg

Ingredients:

- 6 cloves garlic, chopped
- 1/4 teaspoons salt
- 12 cups of water
- 6 cups carrots, chopped
- 4 tablespoons dried dill weed
- 1/2 pound olive oil

Procedure:

1. Take a medium-sized pot, over high heat; combine the water, carrots, garlic, dill weed, salt, and olive oil.
2. Now, bring to a boil, reduce heat and simmer for 30 minutes or until carrots are soft.
3. Take a blender, puree the soup, return to the pot and simmer for an additional 30 to 45 minutes.
4. Lastly, season with additional dill or garlic if needed.

Servings: 8

Preparation Time: 50 minutes

Ingredients:

- 4 medium carrots, chopped
- 2 small green bell peppers, chopped
- 4 garlic cloves, minced
- 4 tomatoes, chopped
- 2 celery stalks, chopped
- 2 tsps dried thyme
- 2 onions, chopped
- 2 tbsps minced cilantro
- 1/2 tsp cayenne pepper
- 8 cups vegetable broth
- 4 tbsps olive oil
- 2 (31-oz.) cans of black beans

Procedure:

1. First, heat the oil in a pot over medium heat.
2. Then, place in onion, celery, carrots, bell pepper, garlic, and tomatoes.
3. Now, sauté for 5 minutes, stirring often.
4. After that, stir in broth, beans, thyme, salt, and cayenne.

5. Then, bring to a boil, then lower the heat, and simmer for 15 minutes.
6. Now, transfer the soup to a food processor and pulse until smooth.
7. In the end, serve in soup bowls garnished with cilantro.

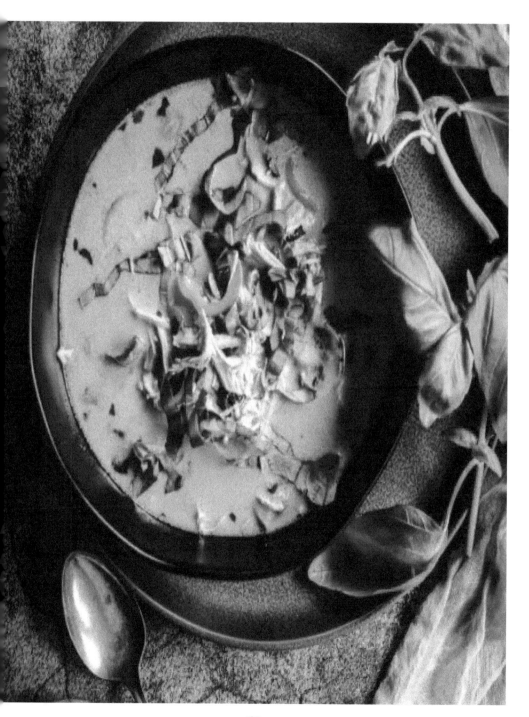

Delicious Basil Coconut Soup

Servings: 8

Preparation Time: 15 minutes

Ingredients:

- 3 garlic cloves, minced
- 2 onions, chopped
- 2 tbsps chopped cilantro
- 3 cups vegetable broth
- 4 tbsps coconut oil
- 8 Lime wedges
- 2 tbsps minced fresh ginger
- 2 cups green bell peppers, sliced
- 2 (13.5-oz.) cans coconut milk
- Juice of 1 lime
- 4 tbsps chopped basil

Procedure:

1. First, warm the coconut oil in a pot over medium heat.
2. Then, place in onion, garlic, and ginger and sauté for 3 minutes.
3. Now, add in bell peppers and broth.
4. After that, bring to a boil, then lower the heat and simmer.

5. Then, stir in coconut milk, lime juice, and chopped cilantro.
6. Now, simmer for 5 minutes.
7. Finally, serve garnished with basil and lime.

Servings: 8

Preparation Time: 25 minutes

Per Serving: Calories: 234; Fat: 5.5g; Carbs: 32.3g; Protein: 14.4g

Ingredients:

- 2 carrots, chopped
- 2 tablespoons olive oil
- 2 parsnips, chopped
- 2 rosemary sprigs, chopped
- Flaky sea salt and ground black pepper, to taste
- 4 tablespoons shallots, chopped
- 32 ounces canned navy beans
- 2 celery stalks, chopped
- 2 teaspoons fresh garlic, minced
- 8 cups vegetable broth
- 4 bay leaves

Procedure:

1. First, in a heavy-bottomed pot, heat the olive over medium-high heat.
2. Now, sauté the shallots, carrot, parsnip, and celery for approximately 3 minutes or until the vegetables are just tender.
3. Then, add in the garlic and continue to sauté for 1 minute or until aromatic.

4. After that, add in the vegetable broth, bay leaves, and rosemary and bring to a boil.
5. Now, immediately reduce the heat to a simmer and let it cook for 10 minutes.
6. Then, fold in the navy beans and continue to simmer for about 5 minutes longer until everything is thoroughly heated.
7. After that, season with salt and black pepper to taste.
8. Finally, ladle into individual bowls, discard the bay leaves and serve hot.

Servings: 6

Preparation Time: 15 minutes

Per Serving: Calories: 154; Fat: 12.3g; Carbs: 9.6g; Protein: 4.4g

Ingredients:

- 2 white onions, chopped
- 2 red bell peppers, chopped
- 1 teaspoon garlic, pressed
- 2 teaspoons Italian herb mix
- 6 cups Cremini mushrooms, chopped
- Sea salt and ground black pepper, to taste
- 2 heaping tablespoons fresh chives, roughly chopped
- 6 tablespoons vegan butter
- 4 tablespoons almond flour
- 6 cups water

Procedure:

1. First, in a stockpot, melt the vegan butter over medium-high heat.
2. Then, once hot, sauté the onion and pepper for about 3 minutes until they have softened.

3. Now, add in the garlic and Cremini mushrooms and continue sautéing until the mushrooms have softened.
4. After that, sprinkle almond meal over the mushrooms and continue to cook for 1 minute or so.
5. Then, add in the remaining ingredients.
6. Now, let it simmer, covered, and continue to cook for 5 to 6 minutes more until the liquid has thickened slightly.
7. Finally, ladle into three soup bowls and garnish with fresh chives.

Servings: 8

Preparation Time: 40 minutes

Per Serving: Calories: 400; Fat: 9g; Carbs: 68.7g; Protein: 13.4g

Ingredients:

- 2 celery stalks, chopped
- 8 large potatoes, peeled and chopped
- 4 garlic cloves, minced
- 4 tablespoons olive oil
- 8 cups vegetable stock
- 2 onions, chopped
- 2 teaspoons fresh basil, chopped
- Salt and fresh ground black pepper, to taste
- 4 tablespoons fresh chives chopped
- 2 teaspoons fresh parsley, chopped
- 2 teaspoons fresh rosemary, chopped
- 2 bays laurel
- 2 teaspoons ground allspice

Procedure:

1. First, in a heavy-bottomed pot, heat the olive oil over medium-high heat.
2. Then, once hot, sauté the onion, celery and potatoes for about 5 minutes, stirring periodically.

3. Now, add in the garlic, basil, parsley, rosemary, bay laurel, and allspice and continue sautéing for 1 minute or until fragrant.
4. After that, add in the vegetable stock, salt, and black pepper and bring to a rapid boil.
5. Then, immediately reduce the heat to a simmer and let it cook for about 30 minutes.
6. Now, puree the soup using an immersion blender until creamy and uniform.
7. Finally, reheat your soup and serve with fresh chives.

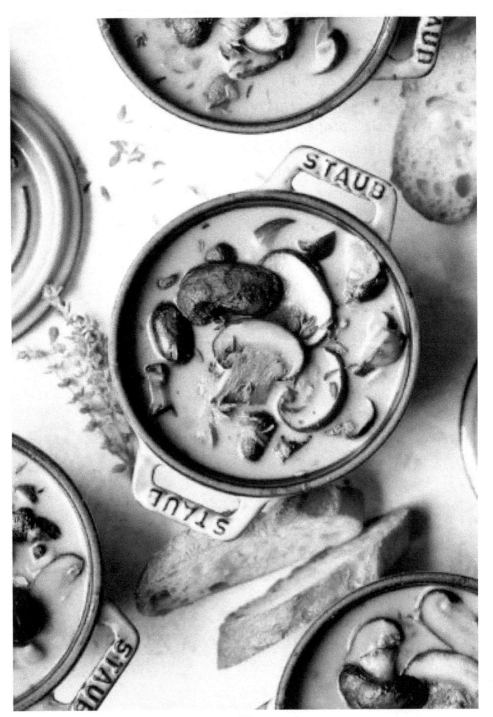

Servings: 6

Preparation Time: 55 minutes

Per Serving: Calories: 313; Fat: 23.5g; Carbs: 14.5g; Protein: 14.5g

Ingredients:

- 2 white onions, chopped
- 6 cloves garlic, minced and divided
- Garlic salt and freshly ground black pepper to seasoned
- 4 sprigs thyme, chopped
- 1 teaspoon red chili flakes
- 6 tablespoons sesame oil
- 4 sprigs rosemary, chopped
- 2 pounds mixed wild mushrooms, sliced
- 1/2 cup flaxseed meal
- 1/2 cup dry white wine
- 6 cups vegetable broth

Procedure:

1. Start by preheating your oven to 395 degrees F.
2. Then, place the mushrooms in a single layer onto a parchment-lined baking pan.
3. Now, drizzle the mushrooms with 1 tablespoon of sesame oil.

4. After that, roast the mushrooms in the preheated oven for about 25 minutes, or until tender.
5. Then, heat the remaining 2 tablespoons of the sesame oil in a stockpot over medium heat.
6. Now, sauté the onion for about 3 minutes or until tender and translucent.
7. After that, add in the garlic, thyme, and rosemary and continue to sauté for 1 minute or so until aromatic.
8. Then, sprinkle a flaxseed meal over everything.
9. Now, add in the remaining ingredients and continue to simmer for 10 to 15 minutes longer or until everything is cooked through.
10. After that, stir in the roasted mushrooms and continue simmering for a further 12 minutes.
11. Finally, ladle into soup bowls and serve hot.

Servings: 5

Preparation Time: 25minutes

Per Serving: Calories: 313; Fat: 23.5g; Carbs: 14.5g;
Protein: 14.5g

Ingredients:

- 2 celeries with leaves, chopped
- 2 carrots, chopped
- 4 garlic cloves, minced
- 2 zucchinis, chopped
- 1 cup Kalamata olives, pitted and sliced
- 4 tablespoons olive oil
- 2 onions, chopped
- 1 teaspoon dried dill
- 10 cups vegetable broth
- 4 medium-sized tomatoes, pureed
- 2,1/2 pounds green beans, trimmed and cut into
  bite-sized chunks
- Sea salt and freshly ground black pepper, to taste
- 1 teaspoon cayenne pepper
- 2 teaspoons oregano

Procedure:

1. First, in a heavy-bottomed pot, heat the olive over medium-high heat.
2. Now, sauté the onion, celery, and carrot for about 4 minutes or until the vegetables are just tender.
3. Then, add in the garlic and zucchini and continue to sauté for 1 minute or until aromatic.
4. After that, stir in the vegetable broth, green beans, tomatoes, salt, black pepper, cayenne pepper, oregano, and dried dill; bring to a boil.
5. Now, immediately reduce the heat to a simmer and let it cook for about 15 minutes.
6. Finally, ladle into individual bowls and serve with sliced olives.

MAIN DISHES

Servings: 8

Preparation Time: 15-30 minutes

Per Serving: Calories 290 Fats 6. 2g Carbs 50. 2g Protein 12g

Ingredients:

- 2 shallots, chopped
- 4 tbsps chopped fresh celery
- 2 garlic cloves, minced
- 8 small lettuce leaves for topping
- 2 (30 oz.) cans pinto beans, drained and rinsed
- 4 tbsps whole-wheat flour
- 2 cups quick-cooking quinoa
- 1 cup tofu mayonnaise for topping
- 1/2 cup chopped fresh basil
- 2 tbsps olive oil
- 4 tbsps pure maple syrup
- Salt and black pepper to taste
- 8 whole-grain hamburger buns, split

Procedure:

1. First, cook the quinoa with 2 cups of water in a medium pot until the liquid is absorbed for about 10 to 15 minutes.

2. Meanwhile, heat the olive oil in a medium skillet over medium heat and sauté the shallot, celery, and garlic until softened and fragrant, 3 minutes.
3. Then, transfer the quinoa and shallot mixture to a medium bowl and add the pinto beans, flour, basil, maple syrup, salt, and black pepper.
4. Mash and mold 4 patties out of the mixture and set aside.
5. After that, heat a grill pan to medium heat and lightly grease with cooking spray.
6. Now, cook the patties on both sides until light brown, compacted, and cooked through, 10 minutes.
7. Then, place the patties between the burger buns and top with the lettuce and tofu mayonnaise.
8. Finally, serve warm.

Servings: 8

Preparation Time: 15-30 minutes

Per Serving: Calories 412 Fats 38. 14g Carbs 13. 19g Protein 6. 57g

Ingredients:

- 2 (20 oz.) can cream of mushroom soup
- 2 tbsps olive oil
- 2 cups tofu mayonnaise
- 1,1/2 cups whole-wheat bread crumbs
- 2 medium red onions, chopped
- 4 cups broccoli florets
- 4 cups grated plant-based cheddar cheese
- 6 tbsps plant butter, melted
- Salt and black pepper to taste
- 6 tbsps coconut cream

Procedure:

1. Start by preheating the oven to 350 F.
2. Then, heat the olive oil in a medium skillet and sauté the broccoli florets until softened, 8 minutes.
3. Now, turn the heat off and mix in the mushroom soup, mayonnaise, salt, black pepper, coconut cream, and onion.
4. After that, spread the mixture into the baking sheet.

5. Then, in a small bowl, mix the breadcrumbs with the plant butter and evenly distribute the mixture on top.
6. Now, add the cheddar cheese and bake the casserole in the oven until golden on top and the cheese melts.
7. Finally, remove the casserole from the oven; allow cooling for 5 minutes, dish, and serve warm.

Servings: 8

Preparation Time: 15-30 minutes

Ingredients:

For the pizza crust:

- 2 tsps yeast
- 6 cups whole-wheat flour
- 6 tbsps olive oil
- 2 cups of warm water
- 2 tsps salt
- 2 pinch sugar

For the topping:

- 1 cup fresh baby spinach
- 1 medium onion, sliced
- 4 tsps dried oregano
- 20 cremini mushrooms, sliced
- 2 cups hummus
- 1 cup cherry tomatoes halved
- 1 cup sliced Kalamata olives

Procedure:

1. First, preheat the oven the 350 F and lightly grease a pizza pan with cooking spray.

2. Take a medium bowl, mix the flour, nutritional yeast, salt, sugar, olive oil, and warm water until smooth dough forms.
3. Allow rising for an hour or until the dough doubles in size.
4. Now spread the dough on the pizza pan and apply the hummus to the dough.
5. Then add the mushrooms, spinach, tomatoes, olives, onion, and top with the oregano.
6. Now bake the pizza for 20 minutes or until the mushrooms soften.
7. In the end, remove from the oven, cool for 5 minutes, slice, and serve.

Homemade Chickpea Burgers with Guacamole

Servings: 8

Preparation Time: 15-30 minutes

Per Serving: Calories 369 kcal Fats 12. 7g Carbs 52. 7g Protein 15. 6g

Ingredients:

For the guacamole:

- 2 tomatoes, chopped
- 2 large avocadoes, pitted and peeled
- 2 small red onions, chopped

For the burgers:

- 4 tbsps quick-cooking oats
- 1/2 cup chopped fresh parsley
- 6 (30 oz.) cans chickpeas, drained and rinsed
- 1/4 tsp black pepper
- 8 whole-grain hamburger buns, split
- 4 tbsps almond flour
- 2 tbsps hot sauce
- 2 garlic cloves, minced
- 1/2 tsp garlic salt

Procedure:

1. First, in a medium bowl, mash avocados and mix in the tomato, onion, and parsley.
2. Then, set aside.
3. Now, in a medium bowl, mash the chickpeas and mix in the almond flour, oats, parsley, hot sauce, garlic, garlic salt, and black pepper.
4. After that, mold 4 patties out of the mixture and set them aside.
5. Then, heat a grill pan to medium heat and lightly grease with cooking spray.
6. Now, cook the bean patties on both sides until light brown and cooked through, 10 minutes.
7. Finally, place each patty between each burger bun and top with the guacamole.

Servings: 8

Preparation Time: 15-30 minutes

Per Serving: Calories 1290 Fats 131. 8g Carbs 15. 2g Protein 24. 4g

Ingredients:

For the stew:

- Salt and black pepper to taste
- 2 tsps chili powder
- 2 tsps onion powder
- 2 tsps cumin powder
- 2 lbs seitan, cut into cubes
- 4 tbsps olive oil
- 2 tsps garlic powder
- 2 limes, juiced
- 2 yellow onions, chopped
- 4 celery stalks, chopped
- 6 green chilies, deseeded and chopped
- 8-10 cloves garlic
- 2 cups vegetable broth
- 2 cups of water
- 2 tsps oregano
- 2 cups chopped tomatoes
- 4 carrots diced

For the brown rice:

- 2 cups of water
- Salt to taste
- 2 cups of brown rice

Procedure:

1. First, heat the olive oil in a large pot, season the seitan with salt, black pepper, and cook in the oil until brown, 10 minutes.
2. Then, stir in the chili powder, onion powder, cumin powder, garlic powder, and cook until fragrant, 1 minute.
3. Now, mix in the onion, celery, carrots, garlic, and cook until softened.
4. After that, pour in the vegetable broth, water, oregano, tomatoes, and green chilies.
5. Then, cover the pot and cook until the tomatoes soften and the stew reduces by half, 10 to 15 minutes.
6. Now, open the lid, adjust the taste with salt, black pepper, and mix in the lime juice.
7. After that, dish the stew and serve warm with the brown rice.
8. Meanwhile, as the stew cooks, add the brown rice, water, and salt to a medium pot.
9. Finally, cook over medium heat until the rice is tender and the water absorbs 15 to 20 minutes.

Servings: 8

Preparation Time: 15-30 minutes

Per Serving: Calories 394 kcal Fats 7. 7g Carbs 73. 9g
Protein 10. 2g

Ingredients:

- 2 medium onions, chopped
- 2 tsps red chili powder
- 8 medium potatoes, peeled and diced
- Salt and black pepper to taste
- 2 cups fresh green peas
- 2 tsps fresh ginger-garlic paste
- 4 tbsps olive oil
- 2 tsps cumin powder
- 1/2 tsp turmeric powder

Procedure:

1. First, steam potatoes in a safe microwave bowl for
   8-10 minutes or until softened.
2. Then, heat the olive oil in a wok and sauté the
   onion until softened, 3 minutes.
3. Now, mix in the chili powder, ginger-garlic paste,
   cumin powder, turmeric powder, salt, and black
   pepper.

4. After that, cook until the fragrant releases, 1 minute.
5. Then, stir in the green peas, potatoes, and cook until softened, 2 to 3 minutes.
6. Finally, serve warm.

Servings: 8

Preparation Time: 15-30 minutes

Per Serving: Calories 354 kcal Fats 20. 8g Carbs 17. 7g
Protein 25. 2g

Ingredients:

For the sauce:

- 1 tsp freshly grated ginger
- 4 tsps cornstarch
- 2/3 tsp allspice
- 6 garlic cloves, minced
- 4 tsps olive oil
- 4 tbsps cold water
- 2/3 tsp red chili flakes
- 1 cup low-sodium soy sauce
- 1 cup + 4 tbsps pure date sugar

For the crisped seitan:

- 2 lbs seitan, cut into 1-inch pieces
- 3 tbsps olive oil

For topping:

- 2 tbsps sliced scallions
- 2 tbsps toasted sesame seeds

Procedure:

1. First, heat the olive oil in a wok and sauté the ginger and garlic until fragrant, 30 seconds.
2. Then, mix in the red chili flakes, Chinese allspice, soy sauce, and date sugar.
3. Now, allow the sugar to melt and set aside.
4. After that, in a small bowl, mix the cornstarch and water.
5. Then, stir the cornstarch mixture into the sauce and allow thickening for 1 minute.
6. Now, turn the heat off.
7. After that, heat the olive oil in a medium skillet over medium heat and fry the seitan on both sides until crispy, 10 minutes,
8. Then, mix the seitan into the sauce and warm over low heat.
9. Now, dish the food, garnish with sesame seeds and scallions.
10. Finally, serve warm with brown rice.

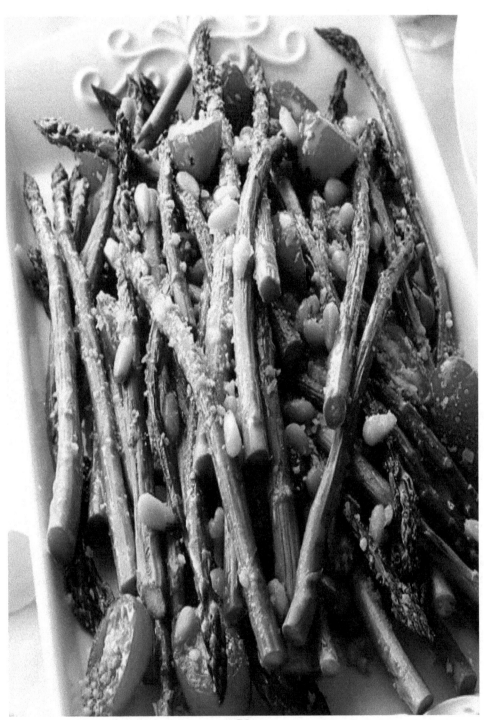

Homemade Baked Potatoes & Asparagus & Pine Nuts

Servings: 8

Preparation Time: 50 minutes

Ingredients:

- 4 tbsps olive oil
- 4 garlic cloves, minced
- 10 cups fresh baby spinach
- Salt and black pepper to taste
- 1 cup ground pine nuts
- 1 cup vegetable broth
- 4 tbsps nutritional yeast
- 2 tsps dried basil
- 2 bunches of asparagus, sliced
- 1 tsp dried thyme
- 4 potatoes, sliced

Procedure:

1. Start by preheating the oven to 370 F.
2. Then, heat half of the oil in a skillet over medium heat.
3. Now, place in garlic, spinach, salt, and pepper and cook for 4 minutes until the spinach wilts.
4. After that, add in basil and thyme.
5. Then, set aside.

6. Now, arrange half of the potato slices on a greased casserole and season with salt and pepper.
7. After that, top with the asparagus slices and finish with the spinach mixture.
8. Then, cover with the remaining potato slices.
9. Now, whisk the broth with nutritional yeast in a bowl.
10. Then, pour over the vegetables. Sprinkle with remaining oil and pine nuts.
11. After that, cover with foil and bake for 40 minutes.
12. Now, uncover and bake for another 10 minutes until golden brown.
13. Finally, serve warm.

Traditional Italian Potato & Swiss Chard Au Gratin

Servings: 8

Preparation Time: 1 h 15 minutes

Ingredients:

- 2 cups Swiss chard, chopped
- 6 tbsps olive oil
- 2 tsps Italian seasoning
- 2 medium yellow onions, minced
- 6 garlic cloves, minced
- 4 tbsps plant-based Parmesan
- Salt and black pepper to taste
- 4 lbs new potatoes, unpeeled, sliced

Procedure:

1. Start by preheating the oven to 360 F.
2. Then, warm half of the oil in a skillet over medium heat.
3. Now, place in onion and garlic and sauté for 3 minutes until translucent.
4. After that, add in Swiss chard to wilt for 3-4 minutes.
5. Then, season with salt and pepper.
6. Now, set aside.
7. After that, arrange half of the potato slices on a greased baking dish.

8. Then, sprinkle with Italian seasoning, salt, and pepper.
9. Now, sprinkle with the remaining olive oil.
10. After that, top with Swiss chard mixture and cover with the remaining potatoes.
11. Then, cover with foil and bake for 1 hour.
12. Now, scatter Parmesan cheese over and bake for another 10 minutes.
13. Finally, serve immediately.

Homemade Sautéed Veggies with Rice

Servings: 8

Preparation Time: 40 minutes

Ingredients:

- 2 medium red bell peppers, chopped
- 4 tbsps olive oil
- 8 shallots, chopped
- 3 cups brown rice, rinsed
- 4 cups corn kernels
- 6 tbsps chopped parsley
- 4 tomatoes, chopped
- 2 medium zucchini, chopped
- 4 cups cooked shelled edamame

Procedure:

1. First, boil 3 cups of salted water in a pot over high heat.
2. Then, place in rice, lower the heat and cook for 20 minutes.
3. Now, set aside.
4. After that, heat the oil in a skillet over medium heat.
5. Then, add in shallots, zucchini, and bell pepper, and sauté for 5 minutes until tender.

6. Now, mix in edamame, corn, tomatoes, salt, and pepper.
7. After that, cook for 5 minutes, stirring often.
8. Now, put in cooked rice and parsley, toss to combine.
9. Finally, serve warm.

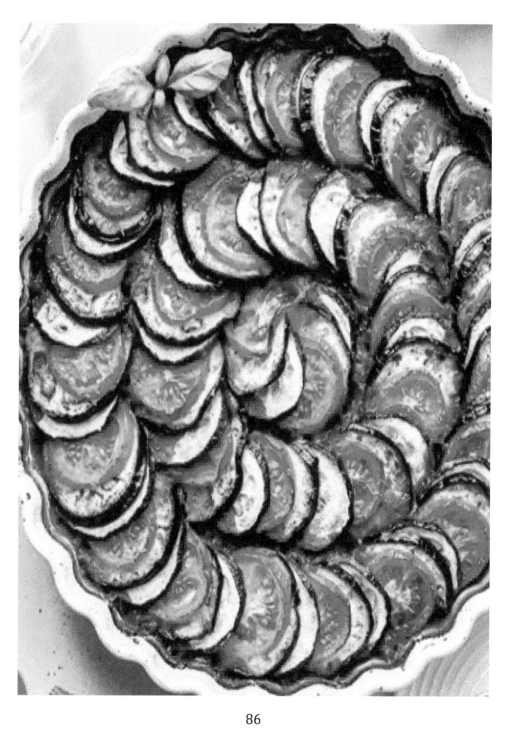

Servings: 12

Preparation Time: 75 minutes

Ingredients:

- 6 tbsps olive oil
- 4 eggplants, sliced diagonally
- 2 onions, chopped
- 4 potatoes, sliced
- 6 garlic cloves, minced
- 6 cups spinach, chopped
- 1,1/2 cups breadcrumbs
- 4 cups kale, chopped
- 6 tbsps plant-based Parmesan
- 4 cups collard greens, chopped
- 2 cups loosely packed basil leaves
- 12 ripe plum tomatoes, sliced

Procedure:

1. Start by preheating the oven to 390 F.
2. Then, arrange the potato slices on a greased baking sheet and the eggplant slices in a separate baking sheet.
3. Now, sprinkle the vegetables with oil, salt, and pepper.
4. After that, cake the eggplants for 10 minutes and the potato for 20 minutes.

5. Then, set aside.
6. Now, heat oil in a skillet over medium heat.
7. After that, place in onion and garlic and sauté for 3 minutes until soft.
8. Then, add in spinach, kale, collard greens, salt, and pepper.
9. Now, cook for 7 minutes until the greens wilt.
10. After that, remove the mixture into a blender.
11. Then, add in basil and remaining oil, salt, and pepper and blend until smooth.
12. Now, on a grease baking dish, arrange half of the potato slices and cover with some greens mixture.
13. After that, add a layer of eggplant slices and cover with more greens mixture.
14. Then, add a layer of tomato slices and cover with more greens mixture.
15. Now, repeat the process until no ingredients are left.
16. After that, sprinkle each layer with salt and pepper.
17. Then, scatter with breadcrumbs and Parmesan cheese.
18. Now, sprinkle the remaining oil.
19. After that, bake for another 10 minutes.
20. Finally, serve warm.

Servings: 8

Preparation Time: minutes

Ingredients:

- 4 sweet potatoes, chopped
- 2 cups green beans, chopped
- 4 cups vegetable broth
- 4 tbsps olive oil
- 2 onions, finely chopped
- 2 cups buckwheat groats

Procedure:

1. Start by preheating the oven to 420 F.
2. Then, arrange the sweet potatoes on a greased baking dish and coat with half of the oil.
3. After that, sprinkle with salt and pepper.
4. Now, roast for 25 minutes, turning once. Set aside.
5. After that, heat the remaining oil in a skillet over medium heat.
6. Then, place the onion and sauté for 3 minutes, stirring often.
7. Now, stir in buckwheat groats and broth.
8. After that, bring to a boil, then lower the heat and simmer for 15 minutes.
9. Then, mix in green beans, sweet potatoes, salt, and pepper.
10. Finally, serve right away.

Servings: 12

Preparation Time: 25 minutes

Per Serving: Calories: 169; Fat: 9.1g; Carbs: 21g; Protein: 1.1g

Ingredients:

- 1/2 cup extra-virgin olive oil
- 2 teaspoons dried oregano
- 2 pounds yam, peeled and cut into 1/8-inch-thick slices
- Sea salt and ground black pepper, to taste
- 1 teaspoon cayenne pepper
- 2 teaspoons dried basil

Procedure:

1. First, toss the yam slices with the remaining ingredients.
2. Then, arrange the yam slices in a single layer on a parchment-lined baking pan.
3. In the end, bake at 400 degrees F for about 20 minutes or until golden and crisp.

SIDE DISHES & SNACKS

Servings: 4

Preparation Time: 10 minutes

Per Serving: Calories291, Total Fat 8. 3g, Saturated Fat 6. 2g, Cholesterol 0mg, Sodium 987mg, Total Carbohydrate 39. 8g, Dietary Fiber 17. 4g, Total Sugars 5. 8g, Protein 16. 5g

Ingredients:

- 1 cup broccoli
- 2 teaspoons garlic powder
- 2 tablespoons coconut oil
- 2 small onions, diced
- 2 lemons, zest, and juice
- 2 cups vegetable broth
- 1 teaspoon kosher salt
- 1 carrot, diced
- 1 cup spinach, chopped
- Ground black pepper to taste
- 1 teaspoon crushed red pepper flakes, or to taste
- 1 cup green lentils
- 1 cup diced tomatoes

Procedure:

1. First, select the Sauté setting on the Instant Pot, add coconut oil and stir onions and carrots, and

broccoli in the hot oil until softened, about 2 minutes.

2. Then, add garlic powder, kosher salt, black pepper, and red pepper flakes; cook and stir to coat for 1 minute.
3. Now, stir lentils, tomatoes, and their juice, and vegetable broth into the onion mixture.
4. After that, lock the lid into place.
5. Then, select Pressure Cook or Manual, and adjust the pressure to High and the time to 12 minutes.
6. After cooking, let the pressure release naturally for 10 minutes, then quickly release any remaining pressure.
7. Then, add spinach, lemon zest, and lemon juice; cook until spinach is wilted, about 5 minutes.
8. Finally, Season with salt and black pepper.

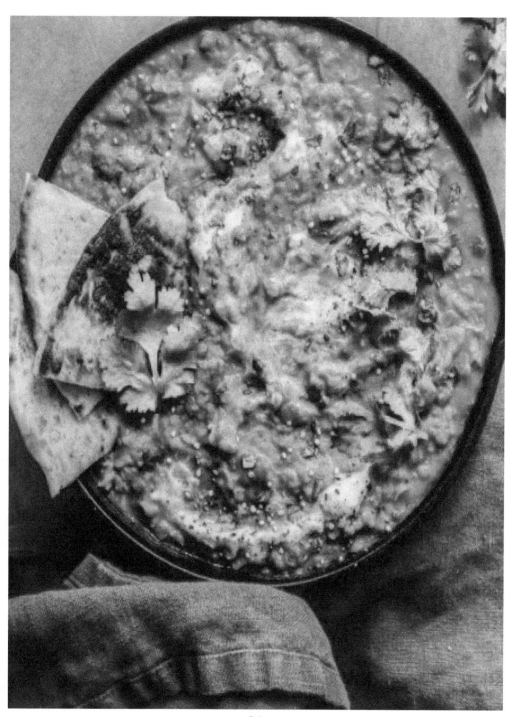

Servings: 4

Preparation Time: 10 minutes

Per Serving: Calories 171, Total Fat 6. 5g Saturated Fat 3. 8g, Cholesterol 15mg, Sodium 700mg, Total Carbohydrate 20. 3g, Dietary Fiber 8. 8g, Total Sugars 2. 7g, Protein 7. 9g

Ingredients:

- 1/2 cup dry brown lentils
- 1/2 cup dry red lentils
- 4 cups of water
- 10 whole garlic cloves
- 1/2 teaspoon salt
- ½ teaspoon ground coriander
- 1/2 teaspoon cayenne pepper, or to taste
- 1/4 teaspoon turmeric powder
- 2 tablespoons butter
- 2 small onion, sliced
- 1 teaspoon cumin seeds
- 1/4 cup soy milk

Procedure:

1. First, soak brown and red lentils in ample cool water for 1 hour to overnight.
2. Then, drain and rinse.

3. Now, select the Sauté setting on the Instant Pot, add butter and stir onions, and cook, often stirring until they turn golden brown.
4. After that, stir in the cumin seeds, and cook until fragrant, about 1 minute.
5. Then, pour in the water, and then add garlic, salt, ground coriander, turmeric powder, and cayenne pepper.
6. Now, add both lentils.
7. After that, select Pressure Cook or Manual, and adjust the pressure to High and the time to 12 minutes.
8. After cooking, let the pressure release naturally for 10 minutes, and then quickly release any remaining pressure.
9. In the end, stir soy milk into the lentils.

Servings: 4

Preparation Time: 15 minutes

Per Serving: Calories 233, Total Fat 8. 1g Saturated Fat 6g, Cholesterol 0mg, Sodium 733mg, Total Carbohydrate 37. 5g, Dietary Fiber 8. 4g, Total Sugars 17. 7g, Protein 9. 3g

Ingredients:

- 2 cups of tomato paste
- 2 tablespoons coconut oil
- 4 cups of water
- 2 teaspoons ginger powder
- 1/2 cup chopped fresh cilantro
- 2 small onions, chopped
- 1 teaspoon garlic powder
- 1 cup dried black-eyed peas (cowpeas)
- 1 teaspoons salt
- 1 teaspoon cumin powder
- 1 teaspoon paprika

Procedure:

1. First, place black-eyed peas into a large container and cover with several inches of cool water; let it stand for 8 hours to overnight.
2. Then, drain and rinse peas.
3. Now, combine black-eyed peas, onions, tomato paste, coconut oil, cilantro, garlic powder, salt,

cumin, paprika, and ginger powder in an Instant Pot; pour 2 cups of water over the pea mixture.

4. After that, select Pressure Cook or Manual, and adjust the pressure to High and the time to 12 minutes.

5. After cooking, let the pressure release naturally for 10 minutes, and then quickly release any remaining pressure.

6. Finally, serve and enjoy.

Servings: 4

Preparation Time: 15 minutes

Per Serving: Calories 147, Total Fat 1. 4g Saturated Fat 0. 1g, Cholesterol 0mg, Sodium 37mg, Total Carbohydrate 30. 9g, Dietary Fiber 6. 2g, Total Sugars 8. 7g, Protein 6. 8g

Ingredients:

- 1 cup chopped onions
- 2 cups chopped green bell pepper
- 1 cup kale
- 2 cups vegetable broth
- 1 cup chopped leeks
- 2 tablespoons olive oil
- 1 cup black-eyed peas
- 2 cups diced tomatoes
- 1 cup of corn

Procedure:

1. First, select the Sauté setting on the Instant Pot, add olive oil and onions in the Instant Pot, and cook until tender.
2. Then, add the green bell pepper, chopped leek, black-eyed peas, tomatoes, corn, and kale.
3. Now, mix well.
4. After that, pour the vegetable broth.

5. Then, select Pressure Cook or Manual, and adjust the pressure to High and the time to 12 minutes.
6. After cooking, let the pressure release naturally for 10 minutes, and then quickly release any remaining pressure.
7. Then, open the lid.
8. Finally, serve and enjoy.

Servings: 4

Preparation Time: 15 minutes

Per Serving: Calories 409, Total Fat 4. 3g Saturated Fat 2. 1g, Cholesterol 8mg, Sodium 567mg, Total Carbohydrate 71g, Dietary Fiber 17. 9g, Total Sugars 7. 7g, Protein 21. 9g

Ingredients:

- 2 red onions
- 1 teaspoon garlic powder
- 4 cups reduced-sodium vegetable broth
- 3 cups dry pinto beans
- 2 bay leafs
- 1 tablespoon butter
- Freshly cracked pepper
- 1 cup diced tomatoes

Procedure:

1. First, add butter, onion, garlic powder, pinto beans, bay leaves, pepper, and broth to the pot, stir briefly to combine, and then place the lid on the Instant Pot.
2. Then, close the steam valve, press the Manual button, select High pressure, then press the + button to increase the time to 35 minutes.
3. Now, allow the pinto beans to cook through the 35-minute cycle.

4. Then, let the pressure release naturally (you'll know, the pressure has been released when the silver float valve has fallen back down and is no longer flush with the top of the lid).
5. After that, once the pressure has been released, open the steam valve and then remove the lid.
6. Then, discard the bay leaf.
7. Now, add the diced tomatoes with all their juices, and then stir to combine.
8. Then, press the Cancel button to Cancel the "keep warm" function, then press the Sauté button and use the Adjust button to select the "Normal" heat level.
9. Let the mixture simmer, often stirring until the beans are very tender and the liquid has thickened.
10. Finally, serve and enjoy.

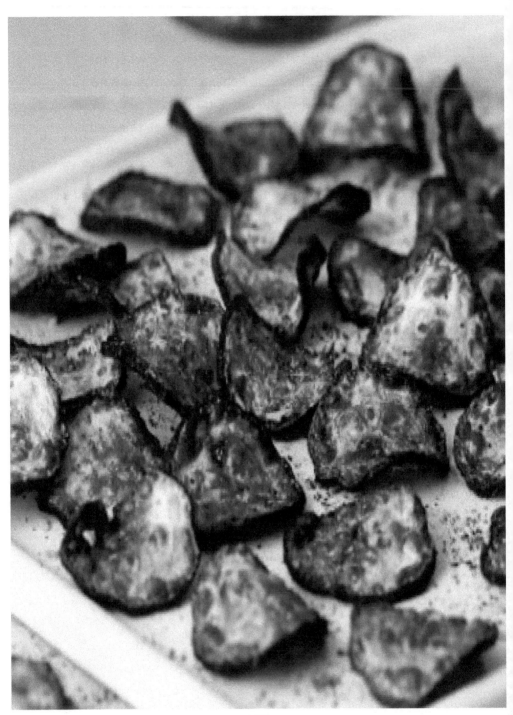

103

Servings: 8

Preparation Time: 26 minutes

Ingredients:

- 3 cups coconut oil
- 2 large yellow squashes
- 2 tbsps taco seasoning

Procedure:

1. First, with a mandolin slicer, cut the squash into thin, round slices and place it in a colander.
2. Then, sprinkle the squash with a lot of salt and allow sitting for 5 minutes.
3. After, press the water out of the squash and pat dry with a paper towel.
4. Now, pour the coconut oil into a deep skillet and heat the oil over medium heat.
5. Then, carefully add the squash slices in the oil, about 20 pieces at a time, and fry until crispy and golden brown.
6. After that, use a slotted spoon to remove the squash onto a paper towel-lined plate.
7. In the end, sprinkle the slices with taco seasoning and serve.

Servings: 8

Preparation Time: 50 minutes

Ingredients:

- 2/3 cup sesame seeds
- 1/2 cup plant butter, melted
- 2/3 cup chia seeds
- 2/3 cup pumpkin seeds
- 2/3 cup sunflower seeds
- 2/3 cup coconut flour

Procedure:

1. Start by preheating the oven to 300 F and line a baking sheet with parchment paper.
2. Then, in a bowl, mix the coconut flour, sesame seeds, sunflower seeds, chia seeds, pumpkin seeds, and salt.
3. Now, add the plant butter, 1 cup of boiling water, and mix until well combined.
4. After that, spread the mixture on the baking sheet and bake in the oven until the batter is firm, 45 minutes.
5. Now, remove the crackers and allow cooling for 10 minutes.
6. In the end, break the crackers into pieces and serve.

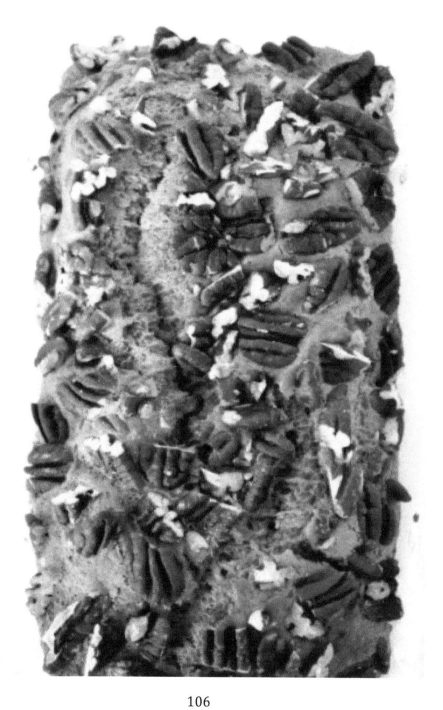

Amazing Pecan Tempeh Cakes

Servings: 8

Preparation Time: 20 minutes

Ingredients:

- 1 cup old-fashioned oats
- Sliced red onion, tomato, lettuce, and avocado
- 8 whole-grain burger buns
- 2 chopped onions
- 4 garlic cloves, minced
- 2 tbsps Dijon mustard
- 1,1/2 cups chopped pecans
- 16 oz. tempeh, chopped
- 2 tbsps minced fresh parsley
- 1 tsp dried oregano
- 1 tsp dried thyme
- Salt and black pepper to taste
- 6 tbsps olive oil

Procedure:

1. First, place the tempeh in a pot with hot water.
2. Then, cook for 30 minutes. Drain and let cool.
3. After that, in a blender, add onion, garlic, tempeh, pecans, oats, parsley, oregano, thyme, salt, and pepper.
4. Now, pulse until everything is well combined.
5. Finally, form the mixture into 4 balls; flatten to make burgers.

Servings: 4

Preparation Time: 15 minutes

Ingredients:

- 4 tbsps pure maple syrup
- 1/2 cup chopped fresh parsley
- 2 lbs baby carrots
- 4 tbsps plant butter
- 2 tbsps freshly squeezed lemon juice
- 1 tsp black pepper

Procedure:

1. First, boil some water in a medium pot.
2. Then, add some salt and cook the carrots until tender, 5 to 6 minutes.
3. Now, drain the carrots.
4. After that, melt the butter in a large skillet and mix in the maple syrup and lemon juice.
5. Now, toss in the carrots, season with black pepper, and toss in the parsley.
6. Finally, serve the carrots.

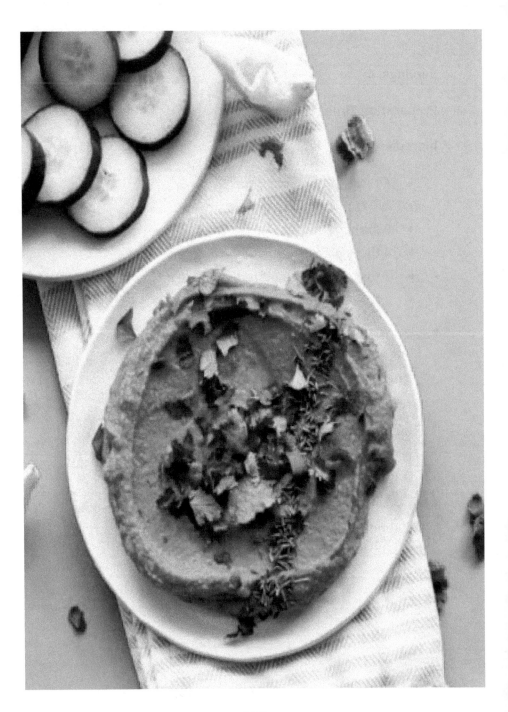

Servings: 20

Preparation Time: 10 minutes

Ingredients:

- 1/2 cup tahini
- 1/2 cup olive oil
- 2 limes, freshly squeezed
- 40 ounces canned or boiled chickpeas, drained
- 2 teaspoons garlic, sliced
- 2 teaspoons coriander seeds
- 1/2 cup chickpea liquid, or more, as needed
- 4 tablespoons fresh cilantro, roughly chopped
- 1/2 teaspoon turmeric
- 1 teaspoon cumin powder
- 2 teaspoons curry powder

Procedure:

1. First, blitz the chickpeas, garlic, tahini, olive oil, lime, turmeric, cumin, curry powder, and coriander seeds in your blender or food processor.
2. Then, blend until your desired consistency is reached, gradually adding the chickpea liquid.
3. Now, place in your refrigerator until ready to serve.
4. After that, garnish with fresh cilantro.
5. Finally, serve with naan bread or veggie sticks, if desired.

Servings: 20

Preparation Time: 55 minutes

Per Serving: Roasted Carrot and Bean Dip

Ingredients:

- 8 tablespoons tahini
- 16 ounces canned cannellini beans, drained
- 2 teaspoons garlic, chopped
- 1 teaspoon dried dill
- 3 pounds carrots, trimmed
- 4 tablespoons olive oil
- 1/2 cup pepitas, toasted
- 4 tablespoons lemon juice
- 4 tablespoons soy sauce
- Sea salt and ground black pepper, to taste
- 1 teaspoon paprika

Procedure:

1. Begin by preheating your oven to 390 degrees F.
2. Then, line a roasting pan with parchment paper.
3. Now, toss the carrots with the olive oil and arrange them on the prepared roasting pan.
4. After that, roast the carrots for about 50 minutes or until tender.
5. Then, transfer the roasted carrots to the bowl of your food processor.

111

6. Now, add in the tahini, beans, garlic, lemon juice, soy sauce, salt, black pepper, paprika, and dill.
7. Then, process until your dip is creamy and uniform.
8. In the end, garnish with toasted pepitas and serve with dippers of choice.

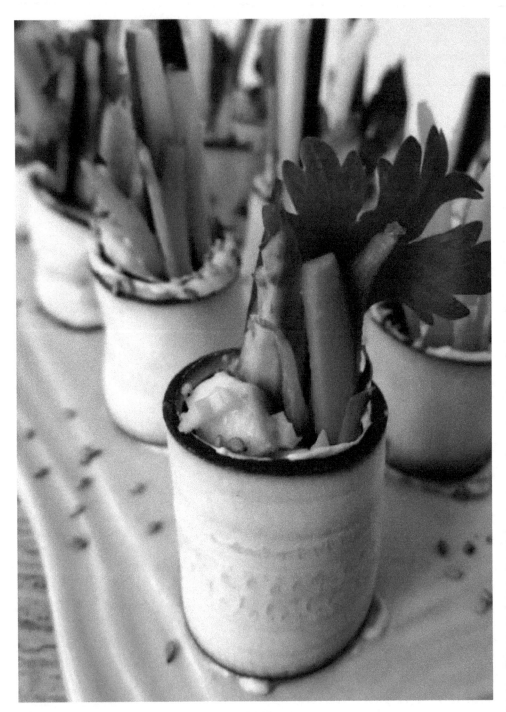

Servings: 10

Preparation Time: 10 minutes

Per Serving: Calories: 129; Fat: 6.3g; Carbs: 15.9g; Protein: 2.5g

Ingredients:

- 2 cups rice, cooked
- 2 small onions, grated
- 2 medium zucchini, cut into strips
- Wasabi sauce, to serve
- 2 carrots, grated
- 2 avocadoes, chopped
- 2 garlic cloves, minced
- Sea salt and ground black pepper, to taste

Procedure:

1. First, in a mixing bowl, thoroughly combine the rice, carrot, onion, avocado, garlic, salt, and black pepper.
2. Then, divide the filling between the zucchini strips and spread it out evenly.
3. Finally, roll the zucchini up and serve with Wasabi sauce.

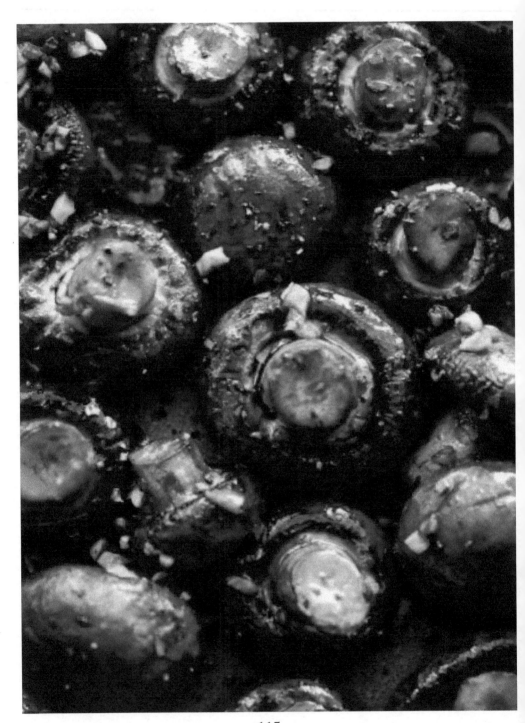

Servings: 8

Preparation Time: 20 minutes

Per Serving: Calories: 136; Fat: 10.5g; Carbs: 7.6g; Protein: 5.6g

Ingredients:

- 6 garlic cloves, minced
- 1 teaspoon dried rosemary
- 6 tablespoons olive oil
- 2 teaspoons dried oregano
- 2 teaspoons dried basil
- Kosher salt and ground black pepper, to taste
- 3 pounds button mushrooms, cleaned

Procedure:

1. First, toss the mushrooms with the remaining ingredients.
2. Then, arrange the mushrooms on a parchment-lined roasting pan.
3. Now, bake the mushrooms in the preheated oven at 420 degrees F for about 20 minutes or until tender and fragrant.
4. Finally, arrange the mushrooms on a serving platter and serve with cocktail sticks.